TRENDS IN SOUTHEAST ASIA

The **ISEAS – Yusof Ishak Institute** (formerly Institute of Southeast Asian Studies) is an autonomous organization established in 1968. It is a regional centre dedicated to the study of socio-political, security, and economic trends and developments in Southeast Asia and its wider geostrategic and economic environment. The Institute's research programmes are grouped under Regional Economic Studies (RES), Regional Strategic and Political Studies (RSPS), and Regional Social and Cultural Studies (RSCS). The Institute is also home to the ASEAN Studies Centre (ASC), the Singapore APEC Study Centre and the Temasek History Research Centre (THRC).

ISEAS Publishing, an established academic press, has issued more than 2,000 books and journals. It is the largest scholarly publisher of research about Southeast Asia from within the region. ISEAS Publishing works with many other academic and trade publishers and distributors to disseminate important research and analyses from and about Southeast Asia to the rest of the world.

COMMUNICATING COVID-19 EFFECTIVELY IN MALAYSIA

Challenges and Recommendations

Serina Rahman

ISSUE
3
2022

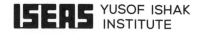 YUSOF ISHAK
INSTITUTE

Published by: ISEAS Publishing
                  30 Heng Mui Keng Terrace
                  Singapore 119614
                  publish@iseas.edu.sg
                  http://bookshop.iseas.edu.sg

ISEAS Library Cataloguing-in-Publication Data

Name(s): Serina Rahman, author.
Title: Communicating COVID-19 effectively in Malaysia : challenges and recommendations / by Serina Rahman.
Description: Singapore : ISEAS-Yusof Ishak Institute, January 2022. | Series: Trends in Southeast Asia, ISSN 0219-3213 ; TRS3/22 | Includes bibliographical references.
Identifiers: ISBN 9789815011319 (soft cover) | ISBN 9789815011326 (pdf)
Subjects: LCSH: Communication in public health—Malaysia. | COVID-19 Pandemic, 2020-—Malaysia.
Classification: LCC DS501 I59T no. 3(2022)

Typeset by Superskill Graphics Pte Ltd
Printed in Singapore by Mainland Press Pte Ltd

FOREWORD

The economic, political, strategic and cultural dynamism in Southeast Asia has gained added relevance in recent years with the spectacular rise of giant economies in East and South Asia. This has drawn greater attention to the region and to the enhanced role it now plays in international relations and global economics.

The sustained effort made by Southeast Asian nations since 1967 towards a peaceful and gradual integration of their economies has had indubitable success, and perhaps as a consequence of this, most of these countries are undergoing deep political and social changes domestically and are constructing innovative solutions to meet new international challenges. Big Power tensions continue to be played out in the neighbourhood despite the tradition of neutrality exercised by the Association of Southeast Asian Nations (ASEAN).

The **Trends in Southeast Asia** series acts as a platform for serious analyses by selected authors who are experts in their fields. It is aimed at encouraging policymakers and scholars to contemplate the diversity and dynamism of this exciting region.

THE EDITORS

Series Chairman:
   Choi Shing Kwok

Series Editor:
   Ooi Kee Beng

Editorial Committee:
   Daljit Singh
   Francis E. Hutchinson
   Norshahril Saat

Communicating COVID-19 Effectively in Malaysia: Challenges and Recommendations

By Serina Rahman

EXECUTIVE SUMMARY

- Malaysia was initially lauded for its ability to combat the first few waves of COVID-19 but infection spikes since the Sabah state elections in September 2020 and subsequent exponential increases in both infections and deaths in 2021 left the nation reeling. Nationwide vaccination is seen as the only way out of the pandemic.
- Malaysia's COVID-19 communication strategy was hampered by political machinations and myriad changes in government. The need to shore up favour among the electorate resulted in inconsistent messaging and regular U-turns whenever there was public outrage at arbitrary restrictions. This resulted in confusion on the ground, preventing successful COVID-19 management and containment.
- Under the current regime, claims to more accessible data have been disputed and doubts have surfaced over data transparency and accuracy. There is an urgent need to ensure convincingly reliable information, as well as to use more engaging messaging on more suitable media.
- A holistic and effective COVID-19 communication strategy should adopt principles from several communication approaches, resulting in messages that are clear, simple and accessible as well as consistent and credible. Audiences should be segmented so that messages can be better tailored to their needs, with adequate information on the necessary steps to prevent infection and spread. Fake news, misinformation, and disinformation should be constantly tackled and debunked.

- The Gerai OA and OA Lindungi Komuniti Facebook pages are outstanding examples of grassroots information dissemination channels that effectively provide fact-checked, coherent and accessible information to local communities in languages and on media best-suited to their audiences.

Communicating COVID-19 Effectively in Malaysia: Challenges and Recommendations

By Serina Rahman[1]

Malaysia first encountered COVID-19 in January 2020 and the crisis has now dragged on for almost two years. Initially lauded for the successful containment of the virus in early 2020, a combination of factors led to a sudden deterioration in conditions. In early 2021, there was a sudden escalation in infections and deaths which peaked in August. Today COVID-19 is being cautiously treated as "endemic" and the economy is slowly reopening given the decline in numbers since August 2021.

For a population of about 32.7 million, positive infection and death rates were relatively high. Total cumulative infections and deaths as at 4 December 2021 stood at 2,643,620 cases and 30,538 deaths respectively. Table 1 indicates the severity of Malaysia's COVID-19 experience in comparison to several other countries.[2]

The country with the closest population to Malaysia is Peru. However, while infection numbers there seem lower than that of Malaysia, deaths are higher. Within the immediate vicinity of Southeast Asia, Malaysia has the highest numbers in terms of deaths and infections. The other countries were cited for their international interest

[1] Serina Rahman is Visiting Fellow in the Malaysia Studies Programme at the ISEAS – Yusof Ishak Institute, Singapore. She is deeply grateful for the input, comments and suggestions by Francis E. Hutchinson, Cassey Lee, Pauline Pooi Yin Leong, and Reita Rahim of Gerai OA for this paper.

[2] Ministry of Health Malaysia CovidNow website, https://covidnow.moh.gov.my/ (accessed 23 November 2021).

Table 1: Comparison of Cumulative COVID-19 Infections and Deaths per Million People (Selected Countries as at 22 November 2021)

Country	Population (2021)	Cumulative Infections		Cumulative Deaths	
		Infections per million people	Estimated % of Population	Deaths per million people	Estimated % of Population
Malaysia	32,776,194	79,066.10	7.91	917.22	0.09
Peru	33,359,418	66,701.32	6.67	6,022.11	0.60
Singapore	5,896,686	46,510.38	4.65	520.13	0.05
Thailand	69,950,850	29,606.63	2.96	292.15	0.03
Indonesia	276,361,783	15,391.41	1.54	520.13	0.05
Philippines	111,046,913	25,456.39	2.55	425.84	0.04
India	1,393,409,038	24,778.42	2.48	334.54	0.03
Saudi Arabia	35,340,683	15,549.16	1.55	249.74	0.02
UK	68,207,116	145,774.52	14.58	2,117.29	0.21
France	65,426,179	112,653.75	11.27	1,788.71	0.18
Italy	60,367,477	81,701.14	8.17	2,207.26	0.22
Russia	145,912,025	63,088.91	6.31	1,784.08	0.18
USA	332,915,073	143,845.01	14.38	2,319.94	0.23
Brazil	213,993,437	102,902.27	10.29	2,863.55	0.29

Note: Figures are deemed underestimates given lack of nationwide COVID-19 testing and possible excess deaths that at time of death cannot be directly attributed to COVID-19. For more information on "excess deaths", refer to *The Economist*, "Tracking Covid-19 excess deaths across countries", https://www.economist.com/graphic-detail/coronavirus-excess-deaths-tracker (accessed 23 November 2021). Countries were selected for this table based on proximity in population (Peru), or location (Southeast Asian countries), or because of international interest or highlight of their COVID-19 situation.

Source: For cumulative COVID-19 figures per million: Our World in Data, https://ourworldindata.org/coronavirus/country/malaysia (accessed 23 November 2021). For country populations: World Population Review, https://worldpopulationreview.com/ (accessed 23 November 2021). Percentages are the author's own calculations.

in the news given their high infections or citizens' unrest in response to COVID-19 restrictions. Other sources note that Malaysia has the fourth highest death rate in Asia, after three Middle Eastern countries.[3] For all of these countries, infection and death numbers are often underreported for myriad reasons.

The number of deaths in Malaysia in the month with the highest mortality (August 2021) alone stood at 7,640; 25.4 per cent of cumulative deaths throughout the 23-month pandemic period. Of the total cumulative deaths, 6,077 (20.2 per cent) were Brought in Dead (BID), meaning that they died outside of a healthcare facility. These figures and widespread images of army field hospitals set up across the country clearly indicate how overburdened the country's healthcare system was over the worst of the pandemic period.

It is broadly understood that an "infodemic" accompanied COVID-19 pandemic woes worldwide. An "infodemic" is defined by the World Health Organization as "an over-abundance of information" that makes it difficult for people to discern fact from fake news, resulting in a lack of accurate knowledge of what to do in the coronavirus crisis.[4] Within this spectrum of false information lies the notion of "disinformation" which is "deliberately propagated false information" and "misinformation" or "false information that may have been unintentionally propagated."[5]

Misinformation, disinformation and conspiracy theories dampened efforts to inform and warn citizens about the severity of the virus, and

---

[3] The Middle Eastern countries that have higher death rates than Malaysia are Iran, Lebanon and Jordan. Refer to *Malaysiakini*, "Covid-19 deaths (Nov 21): 38 reported fatalities, total at 29,978", 21 November 2021, https://www.malaysiakini.com/news/600048 (accessed 23 November 2021).

[4] World Health Organization (WHO), "Novel Coronavirus(2019-nCoV)", *Situation Report -13*, 2 February 2020, https://www.who.int/docs/default-source/coronaviruse/situationreports/20200202-sitrep-13-ncov-v3.pdf

[5] B.H. Spitzberg, "Comprehending Covidiocy Communication: Dis-misinformation, Conspiracy Theory, and Fake News", in *Communicating Science in Times of Crisis: COVID-19 Pandemic*, edited by H.D. O'Hair and M.J. O'Hair (New Jersey: John Wiley and Sons, 2021), p. 17.

some simply refused to adapt their behaviour to prevent infection spread.[6] Malaysia was not exempted from this problem, as the country also faced issues of fake news, vaccine conspiracies and COVID-19 deniers which hampered strategies to mitigate the pandemic.[7]

This paper will attempt to assess the extent to which the government's communication strategies have been effective, and determine the factors driving these strategies. This is especially important given the evolving COVID-19 situation and the ever-present threat of new variants that can prolong the pandemic's impacts.

Malaysia's journey with COVID-19 will first be outlined, then several recommended approaches to crisis communication will be explored. How the Malaysian government's communication effort (through selected primary mediums) has evolved over the course of this pandemic will be examined against a suggested amalgamation of those approaches.

The politics of top-down crisis communication in Malaysia will also be examined as the politicization of the pandemic cannot be segregated from the country's pandemic management. A brief comparison of two ground-up communication initiatives that have worked to provide relevant and accessible content to indigenous communities and provide clarification on the multitude of confusing and overlapping restrictions, protocols and myriad other issues facing the country follows. The paper will end with an examination of the most recent evolution of communication strategies under the latest government regime, and look towards an "endemic" future and economic reopening.

---

[6] Z. Barua, S. Barua, S. Aktar, N. Kabir, and M. Li, "Effects of Misinformation on COVID-19 Individual Responses and Recommendations for Resilience of Disastrous Consequences of Misinformation", *Progress in Disaster Science* 8 (2020), https://doi.org/10.1016/j.pdisas.2020.100119

[7] N. Masngut, and E. Mohamad, "Association between Public Opinion and Malaysian Government Communication Strategies about the Covid-19 Crisis: Content Analysis of Image Repair Strategies in Social Media", *Journal of Medical Internet Research* 23, no. 8 (August 2021), https://doi.org/10.2196/28074

MALAYSIA'S COVID-19 EXPERIENCE

Malaysia was initially successful in suppressing infection numbers after COVID-19 was first detected in the country and a wave of cases after a religious gathering in February 2020. However, case numbers began to surge again after the Sabah state elections in September later that year. This was deemed the third wave, leading to high infection numbers (and many deaths) in Sabah, before spreading to the Klang Valley as politicians and their staff returned from campaigning without proper quarantine procedures or testing.

With many states in the Recovery Movement Control Order (RMCO) phase at the time, some took the opportunity to cross state boundaries for the year-end holiday season even as celebrations were meant to be curtailed and muted. This led to yet another upsurge in infections, and by 11 January 2021, a second Movement Control Order (MCO) was reinstated.

The political decision (publicly announced as "economic need") to leave factories open despite the nationwide lockdown on other business sectors in this phase, led to quick contagion amongst (largely) foreign factory workers. By mid-2021, the COVID-19 infection began to spread to rural areas through locals who also worked in factories and brought the virus back to their communities, including rural and forest-fringing indigenous communities.[8]

A portion of these infections were also the result of those who ignored the Ministry of Health (Kementerian Kesihatan Malaysia, or KKM) warnings and Standard Operating Procedure (SOP) restrictions

---

[8] Refer to Ministry of Finance, "Workplace Clusters Record Highest Covid-19 Cases—Tengku Zafrul", Press Citations, 26 July 2021, https://www.mof.gov. my/en/news/press-citations/workplace-clusters-record-highest-covid-19-cases-tengku-zafrul. However, the Federation of Manufacturers, Malaysia disputes these claims. Bernama, "FMM Clears Misconception about Covid-19 Cases from Factory Clusters", *Edge Markets*, 14 July 2021, https://www.theedgemarkets. com/article/fmm-clears-misconception-covid19-cases-factory-clusters

and crossed state lines for festive occasions, funerals, and weddings.[9] Added to this were those who did not take enough precautions to protect themselves or refused to get vaccinated.

Table 2 traces the key dates throughout this journey and illustrates how many have died in 2021 compared to numbers in 2020. The virus epicentre moved beyond the Klang Valley in the second half of 2021 to other states where vaccination percentages were far lower (given the national vaccination programme's early focus on Labuan, Sarawak, Kuala Lumpur and Selangor).

OVERCOMING THE INFODEMIC WITH A COMBINATION OF COMMUNICATION APPROACHES

The COVID-19 pandemic was a wholly new experience for the world. Uncertainty about its source, cause and infectivity led to a raft of conspiracy theories, unhelpful accusations, and unverified folk cures. This glut of information from the very beginning made it more difficult for health authorities to underscore the need for personal precautions even as they hastened to find out more about the virus and its prevention.

Figure 1 provides a summary of factors that hamper effective communication in times of crisis.[10] As explained at length in O'Hair and O'Hair (2021), *optimism bias* refers to the tendency of an information recipient to believe that he or she is less likely to be personally affected by the pandemic,[11] which is slightly different from those who have *low-*

---

[9] S. Salim, "Health DG: 60 Hari Raya and Gawai Clusters Found, with 3,511 Infections and 20 Deaths", *Edge Markets*, 10 June 2021, https://www.theedgemarkets.com/article/health-dg-60-hari-raya-and-gawai-festive-clusters-found-3511-positive-cases-and-20-deaths

[10] Collated from myriad chapters in *Communicating Science in Times of Crisis: COVID-19 Pandemic*, edited by H.D. O'Hair and M.J. O'Hair (New Jersey: John Wiley and Sons, 2021).

[11] K.B. Wright, "Social Media, Risk Perceptions Related to COVID-19, and Health Outcomes," in *Communicating Science in Times of Crisis*, edited by O'Hair and O'Hair, p. 131.

Table 2: Summary of Key Dates, Infection and Deaths in Malaysia's COVID-19 Experience

Date	Situation	Cumulative Infections (Unless Otherwise Stated)	Cumulative Deaths (Unless Otherwise Stated)
24/01/20	First COVID-19 infection	22 cases up to 15/02/20	0
27/02/20	2nd wave: *Tabligh* cluster	3,370	34
		Figures include international event participants who returned to their home countries	
18/03/20		MCO 1.0—BORDERS CLOSED	
31/07/20	Prior to Sabah elections	Sabah: 397 active cases at this time (8,976 cumulative cases)	125
	January – August 2020	9,340	100 deaths during this period only (127 cumulative deaths)
26/09/20	3rd wave: Sabah state elections	Sabah: 1,547 active cases at this time (10,769 cumulative cases)	133
31/10/20	Post Sabah elections	Sabah: 14,519 active cases at this time (31,548 cumulative cases)	249
	First 9 days of 2021	18,549 new cases during this period only (133,559 cumulative cases)	71 deaths during this period only (542 cumulative deaths)
11/01/21		MCO 2.0—STATE OF EMERGENCY	
01/06/21		MCO 3.0—PHASE 1 OF THE RECOVERY PLAN	
	July 2021 only	354,305 new cases during this period only (1,113,272 cumulative cases)	4,014 dead during this period only (9,024 cumulative deaths)
	August 2021 only *(pandemic peak)*	615,832 new cases during this period only (1,746,254 cumulative cases)	7,640 dead during this period only −1,414 (20%) BID (16,664 cumulative deaths)

Notes: MCO: Movement Control Orders; BID: Brought in dead.
Data sources: Ministry of Health Malaysia's COVID-19 website, https://covid-19.moh.gov.my/

Figure 1: Obstacles to Effective Communication

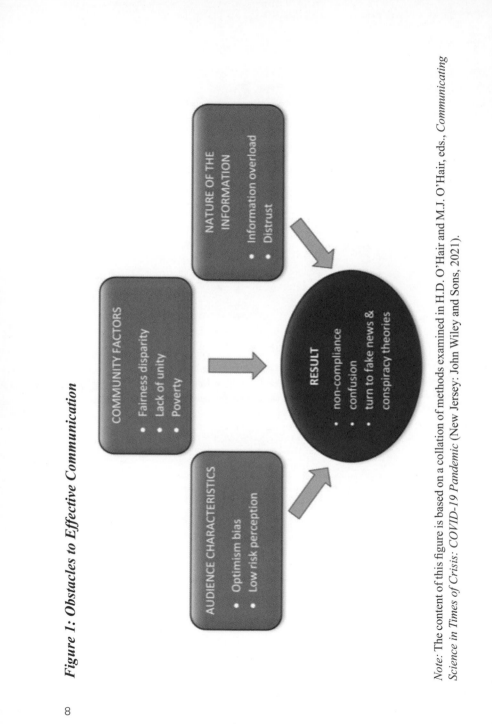

Note: The content of this figure is based on a collation of methods examined in H.D. O'Hair and M.J. O'Hair, eds., *Communicating Science in Times of Crisis: COVID-19 Pandemic* (New Jersey: John Wiley and Sons, 2021).

risk perception. The latter believe that they are not vulnerable to the virus as they are confident that they know how to deal with it.[12] *Fairness disparity* comes about when there are deemed double standards in the enforcement of SOPs, and a *lack of unity* prevents a nation from coming together across myriad divisions to deal with the pandemic.

Poverty tends to inhibit necessary actions to prevent infection because of the need to earn a living, provide food for families and a lack of proper comprehension of the severity of COVID-19. Sometimes a lack of worldly experience and education can result in a *lower cognitive ability* to process an intangible, distant danger such as a virus, especially when larger more immediate needs of survival, food and shelter dominate. *Distrust* occurs when the information (or its source) is deemed to be lacking in integrity, honesty or transparency.

The cumulative effect of all these factors is non-compliance to pandemic SOPs because of confusion and reliance on fake news. This then may have led to more infections that could have otherwise been prevented. It would thus be beneficial to design a cohesive communication strategy that taps several fields, theories and frameworks, as shown in Figure 2 and overcomes the obstacles discussed earlier.

Aspects of science communication enable clear and accessible information to be disseminated to a doubtful audience that needs valid and reliable information to counter uncertainty. Given the severity of the COVID-19 crisis, message recipients need to know how to respond in order to take appropriate action to protect themselves. Because of the extent of the infection and how severely it cripples national healthcare systems and threatens lives, some aspects of terror management could also be useful to ensure better public understanding of the possibility of death because of the virus. Terror management theory examines the handling of "existential anxiety generated by their fear of death and

---

[12] K. Real, K. Hamilton, T. Zborowsky, and D. Gregory, "Communication and COVID-19: Challenges in Evidence-Based Healthcare Design", in *Communicating Science in Times of Crisis*, edited by O'Hair and O'Hair, p. 85.

Figure 2: A Consolidated Approach to COVID-19 Communication Combining Several Methods

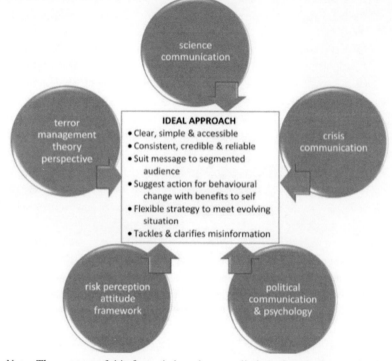

IDEAL APPROACH
- Clear, simple & accessible
- Consistent, credible & reliable
- Suit message to segmented audience
- Suggest action for behavioural change with benefits to self
- Flexible strategy to meet evolving situation
- Tackles & clarifies misinformation

Note: The content of this figure is based on a collation of methods examined in H.D. O'Hair and M.J. O'Hair, eds., *Communicating Science in Times of Crisis: COVID-19 Pandemic* (New Jersey: John Wiley and Sons, 2021).

uncertainty".[13] The theory thus helps communication strategists to devise better ways to reduce anxiety and enable audiences to cope with possible panic and distress during these difficult times.

---

[13] C.H. Miller, and H. Ma, "How Existential Anxiety Shapes Communication in Coping with the Coronavirus Pandemic: A Terror Management Theory Perspective", in *Communicating Science in Times of Crisis*, edited by O'Hair and O'Hair, p. 59.

As discussed in myriad approaches in O'Hair and O'Hair (2021), given that a nationwide problem requires political will and machinery to manage, aspects of *political communication and psychology* to determine who should be seen to be in charge, and whether he or she is deemed credible for that role, makes a difference in pandemic resolution efforts. Unquestionable leadership, reliability and integrity are key to politically driven pandemic management efforts as they directly influence citizens' responses to health advisories and restrictions. The *political environment* also determines who controls the narrative (i.e., accurate medical information and advice being disseminated or fake news taking over). An effective communication strategy will thus consider these factors for better impact.

The *risk perception attitude framework* helps to break down audiences into segregated targets that enable messaging to be specifically designed for each group's attributes. This ensures that messaging resonates with targeted recipients and results in the desired action or behavioural change.

The ideal communication strategy as shown in Figure 2 thus combines useful aspects from each of these approaches, and can provide segmented audiences with clear, accessible and verifiable information that can be related to and accepted for behavioural change so as to prevent widespread infection. Messaging must counter false information head on and be flexible enough to meet inevitable changes in an extremely fluid situation.

MALAYSIA'S COMMUNICATIONS ECOSYSTEM FOR COVID-19

The following sections will examine Malaysia's information ecosystem and use the framework discussed above to analyse selected official communication content disseminated by the KKM throughout the pandemic period.

Notwithstanding myriad changes of government and leadership throughout the pandemic period, there are three main official sources of information: the Prime Minister's Office for overall updates and declarations (usually of pandemic status and offers of aid), the Ministry of Health for medically related information on the virus, and the National Security Council for the necessary responses to the pandemic.

There are, however, multiple other layers of communication. At the state, district or local council levels, restriction orders are broken down into specific SOPs by which the public needs to abide. East Malaysian states have the leeway to decide on their own COVID-19 restrictions, often deviating from federal mandates based on what the state feels is more effective for their local situation.[14] Figure 3 illustrates these main sources of information.

Malaysian citizens and residents receive top-down COVID-19 related information via a mix of official and social media sources. There is a tendency for higher educated urban audiences to tap on more traditional online news media (both international and local) and Twitter, while more rural, less educated audiences tend to depend on social media channels such as WhatsApp and TikTok, as well as traditional television or radio news programmes.[15]

Facebook, YouTube and Telegram seem to be popular with both rural and urban communities, though each will have their own community bubbles depending on their choice of friends and interest groups, which then creates an echo chamber of views that often serve to reinforce their own preconceived ideas of the virus, vaccines and its "cures".[16]

---

[14] This paper will focus mainly on the federal communication content and strategy and will not delve into the details or differences at the state levels. Also refer to the following for more information on East Malaysia's exemptions: *Borneo Post Online*, "CM: Thankfully S'wak Has Powers to Make Decisions Apt to Situation in the State", 21 July 2021, https://www.theborneopost.com/2021/07/21/cm-thankfully-swak-has-powers-to-make-decisions-apt-to-situation-in-the-state/; and T. Yeoh, "Federal-State Friction Amid Malaysia's Dual Political and Pandemic Plight", *New Mandala*, 12 August 2020, https://www.newmandala.org/federal-state-friction-amid-malaysias-dual-political-and-pandemic-plight/

[15] Malaysia Communications and Multimedia Commission, *Internet Users Survey 2018* (Cyberjaya: Government of Malaysia, 2018).

[16] The caveat to this is that Facebook seems to be age-specific, with younger audiences preferring TikTok and Instagram.

Figure 3: COVID-19 Communication Ecosystem in Malaysia

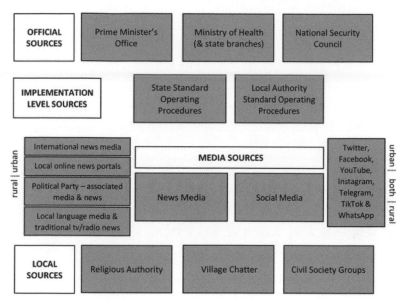

Source: Author's own.

Political, work or education-related divisions between people can be seen in their choices of online news and media consumption. News portals deemed unaligned to the ruling party, and therefore providing "alternative news" compared to government-owned or sanctioned media, such as *Malaysiakini* and the *Malaysian Insight* are more popular with the English-educated, more well-off and vocally political, than rural or lower income groups. Business publications such as the *Edge* also cater to the more elite or educated than the average blue-collar citizen. While this is not a regular source of COVID-19 information, any pandemic-related news printed here might be assumed more credible to its audiences.

Local language media such as *Utusan* (deemed to be aligned with UMNO), *Metro* or *Sinar* (more of a tabloid) are more popular with Malay ethnic communities who eschew "alternative" (deemed "opposition")[17] news portals. Local language news for the Tamil-speaking and ethnic Chinese communities are also more popular beyond primary city centres such as Kuala Lumpur.

There are also other local sources of information that are often deemed more reliable on account of their proximity to their audiences (in terms of social presence, as friends, family, or trusted confidantes). These include local religious authorities or figures, civil society groups that might be regular providers of aid or other assistance, and hearsay from daily community gatherings (at coffeeshops, jetties, rest places and front porches) during the less restrictive phases of the MCO.

The analysis in this paper will be based largely on the Malaysian Ministry of Health (KKM) Facebook pages between January 2020 and September 2021. This medium was selected as it appears to be the main channel through which KKM disseminated information to the masses at the time, even as it also updated its websites with many other details, and replicates some of the graphics from its pages onto the MySejahtera (movement and contact tracing) application. Information from the KKM Facebook pages was often shared on other government Facebook pages, including that of the National Security Council (Majlis Keselamatan Negara, or MKN).[18]

KKM has two Facebook pages: Kementerian Kesihatan Malaysia, which serves as the main social media mouthpiece of the ministry, and Kementerian Kesihatan Malaysia – Portal MyHealth which is run by the Health Education Division (also under KKM), with a focus on providing

---

[17] Given the many changes in government over the past three years, it needs to be explained that the term "opposition" on the ground has always been assigned to parties opposed to UMNO and the Barisan Nasional (BN) coalition. This branding has evolved as a result of more than sixty years of rule of the BN (predominantly UMNO) government.

[18] While the complete communication portfolio by the government encompasses several other channels, this paper will only focus on this one aspect as one of the main mediums of communication with a broad reach. The rest will be analysed in a more complete academic paper which is still work-in-progress.

the latest news, information, and health tips. The Health Education Division is also on Instagram, Twitter and Telegram.

Embedded live and video briefings, PDF press releases and myriad other statistics, data and other information are posted on a number of KKM-related websites depending on who is speaking and what their focus is on. KKM has an official website (https://moh.gov.my) which embeds the official KKM Facebook page on its homepage. When Adham Baba was Health Minister, there was a special COVID-19 website (https://covid-19.moh.gov.my/) that provided the latest (or past) information on the pandemic, searchable by date.

Under the current government, with Khairy Jamaluddin as the new Minister of Health, a new website, *CovidNow* was launched on 9 September 2021 (https://covidnow.moh.gov.my/).[19] However the older COVID-19 website continues to operate and is updated daily with some information being easier to find than on the new *CovidNow* website. The Director-General of Health also has his own website, *From the Desk of the Director-General of Health Malaysia* (https://kpkesihatan.com/), which now seems to focus on posting daily press releases from this office.

Figure 4 illustrates the communication components that will be examined in this paper. The primary focus of this analysis will be on the main KKM Facebook page. Some content from the personal Facebook page of the Director General (DG) of Health, Dr Noor Hisham Abdullah (set as a public "government official" account) will also be raised in comparison to the official pages. Many of the announcements by the Prime Minister or the Head of the National Security Council were made on their official or personal Facebook pages or reposted there from official ministry PDF statements.

A comparison to two ground-up efforts at clarifying and disseminating accurate COVID-19 information through the Gerai OA (OA Shop) and

---

[19] *Sun Daily*, "MOH Launches New Covid-19 Data Website", 9 September 2021, https://www.thesundaily.my/local/moh-launches-new-covid-19-data-website-CC8316721

Figure 4: Malaysia Ministry of Health (KKM) Communication Components and Other Sources

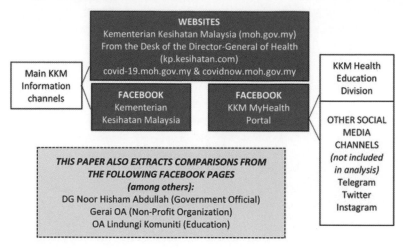

Source: Author's own.

OA Lindungi Komuniti (Indigenous People Protect Our Community) Facebook pages will be done towards the end of this paper.

THE POLITICS OF MALAYSIA'S COVID-19 COMMUNICATION STRATEGY

Malaysia's approach to COVID-19 communication is the "politician prominence model" where a politician demonstrates that he holds the primary decision-making power and communicates those decisions to the public even as he accepts advice from experts.[20]

However, Malaysia's government has been less than stable throughout this extended pandemic period. There have been three governments in

---

[20] D. Lilleker, I.A. Coman, M. Gregor, and E. Novelli, eds., *Political Communication and COVID-19: Governance and Rhetoric in Times of Crisis* (Oxford: Routledge, 2021), p. 3.

power since COVID-19 first appeared in Malaysia, and communication strategies have evolved throughout each regime. Table 3 maps the changes in government with significant phases of the country's pandemic journey.

When COVID-19 was first detected in Malaysia on 24 January 2020, the Pakatan Harapan (PH) government was in power. The virus was little understood then, and it was not yet deemed a national threat, but an external hazard that could be prevented from entering Malaysia. Images on the Malaysian Ministry of Health's Facebook pages showed the then Minister of Health Dr Dzulkefly Ahmad and his deputy inspecting temperature scanners at airport entry points.[21] The minsters were also featured meeting with a few other prominent figures such as then Deputy Prime Minister Dr Wan Azizah Wan Ismail.[22]

The key to the success of the politician-prominence model of communication is the perceived capability of political leaders to deal with a national health crisis. Both Dr Dzulkefly and Dr Wan Azizah are medical doctors, and their combined appearance served to bolster the message that they were coping with the threat of the pandemic based on credible and qualified medical knowledge.

The Tablighi Jamaat religious conference that took place at the Masjid Jamek in Sri Petaling, Kuala Lumpur occurred between 27 February and 1 March. By the time the resultant positive infections from this event appeared (two weeks after the large gathering), the government had changed hands and Muhyiddin Yassin was Prime Minister, with Ismail Sabri Yaakob in charge of the National Security Council and Dr Adham Baba as Minister of Health.

The DG of Health first appeared on the daily briefing post the same day that KKM congratulated Muhyiddin Yassin on his appointment as Prime Minister, perhaps because the Cabinet had not yet been

---

[21] Refer to the KKM Facebook page, https://www.facebook.com/kementerian kesihatanmalaysia/photos/a.10151657414821237/10156673994476237

[22] https://www.facebook.com/kementeriankesihatanmalaysia/photos/a.10151657414821237/10156708204736237

Table 3: Changes in Government Throughout Malaysia's Pandemic Experience

Government in Power	Pandemic Phase	COVID-19 situation
Pakatan Harapan (PM: Mahathir Mohamad Minister of Health: Dzulkefly Ahmad)	First wave	First COVID-19 infection in Malaysia (24 June 2020)
Perikatan Nasional (PM: Muhyiddin Yassin Minister of Health: Adham Baba)	Second wave: Sri Petaling *Tabligh* cluster leading to MCO1.0	First escalation in numbers: 29 accumulated infections; 0 deaths (1 March 2020)
United Malay National Organization (PM: Ismail Sabri Yaakob Minister of Health: Khairy Jamaluddin)	MCO 3.0/Phase 1 of the Recovery Plan	1,535,286 accumulated infections; 13,936 deaths (21 August 2021)

Note: (PM: Prime Minister) - COVID-19 infection numbers sourced from Malaysian Ministry of Health (KKM) website, https://covid-19.moh.gov.my/

Source: Author's own compilation.

appointed.[23] However, after Dr Adham Baba was appointed Minister of Health on 10 March 2021,[24] he overtook prominence on KKM's social media, especially with publicity visits to frontliners and hospitals.

As Malaysia moved into MCO 1.0 and closed its national borders, DG Noor Hisham reappeared on KKM's Facebook page, in an image of him at a press conference updating the nation on the COVID-19 situation.[25] At this point, the official communication strategy had evolved into an "expert appointee prominence model", in which the Minister of Health's role as spokesperson had been relegated to the DG. This was perhaps to increase the credibility of the government pandemic response.[26] This measure seemed to have been taken after several highly publicized gaffes by Dr Adham Baba, for which he was accused of spreading misinformation and widely deemed unqualified for pandemic management on social media.[27]

By 19 May 2020, the DG of Health, Dr Noor Hisham Abdullah announced that five generations of infections had been determined from the religious cluster, with 48 per cent[28] of all infections in the country at the time (1,218 active cases of the 6,978 total accumulated cases, 114 accumulated deaths)[29] traced back to it.

---

[23] https://www.facebook.com/kementeriankesihatanmalaysia/photos/a.10151657414821237/10156786010426237

[24] https://www.facebook.com/kementeriankesihatanmalaysia/photos/a.10151657414821237/10156815596866237

[25] https://www.facebook.com/kementeriankesihatanmalaysia/photos/a.10151657414821237/10156845896151237

[26] Lilleker et al. eds., *Political Communication and COVID-19*, p. 3.

[27] *Malaysiakini*, "Health Minister Gets Roasted for Misinformation over Warm Water Tip", 21 March 2020, https://www.malaysiakini.com/news/515839

[28] *Star Online*, "COVID-19: 972 More Cases Traced Back to Tabligh Cluster", 19 May 2020, https://www.thestar.com.my/news/nation/2020/05/19/covid-19-927-more-cases-traced-back-to-tabligh-cluster

[29] KKM website, https://covid-19.moh.gov.my/terkini/052020/situasi-terkini-19-mei-2020

DG Noor Hisham continued to be the prominent KKM spokesperson, providing daily information on the latest COVID-19 infections and other statistics. On the other hand, the minister and deputy minister were featured on KKM's social media pages during cheque handover events and other ceremonial photo opportunities.[30] Pandemic management credibility clearly rested on the Director-General.

In February 2021, Malaysia began vaccinating its citizens.[31] It was during this time that infection numbers had begun to rise exponentially, and vaccinations were seen as the only hope that Malaysia had to overcome COVID-19. With attention averted to national vaccination rates, then Minister of Science, Technology and Innovation (MOSTI) Khairy Jamaluddin began to gain prominence in COVID-19-related news. A new website for the Special Committee on COVID-19 Vaccine Supply Access (JKJAV) was launched on 1 March 2021 providing vaccination-related information, with regular public updates from the MOSTI minister.

Under the latest regime change in August 2021, Khairy Jamaluddin was reassigned as Minister of Health (Dr Adham Baba became MOSTI minister). His rising popularity and assumed credibility as the result of what was touted as a successful and speedy vaccination programme,[32] carried over into his role at KKM. DG Noor Hisham then seemed to take a backseat again as Khairy Jamaluddin took prominence on KKM's

---

[30] Refer to these posts on the KKM Facebook page, https://www.facebook.com/kementeriankesihatanmalaysia/photos/a.10151657414821237/10156866779116237 (Health Minister at an event); https://www.facebook.com/kementeriankesihatanmalaysia/photos/a.10151657414821237/10156868701396237 (Deputy Health Minister at an event); https://www.facebook.com/kementeriankesihatanmalaysia/photos/a.10151657414821237/10156869562381237 (DG Noor Hisham providing COVID-19 information).

[31] P.P. Kumar, "Malaysia Starts COVID Vaccines in Crucial Week for Asian Jabs", *Nikkei Asia*, 24 February 2021, https://asia.nikkei.com/Spotlight/Coronavirus/Malaysia-starts-COVID-vaccines-in-crucial-week-for-Asian-jabs

[32] N.A. Mohammad Radhi, "Malaysia Tops in Vaccination Rate", *New Straits Times*, 4 August 2021, https://www.nst.com.my/news/nation/2021/08/714696/malaysia-tops-vaccination-rate

social media pages, and as its main spokesperson. The government's communication approach has now returned to the "politician prominence model".

The incessant political drama taking place during a national health crisis seemed to imply that politicians were more interested in retaining or regaining power than dealing with the urgent problems of its desperate citizens. As a result, there was widespread distrust and dissatisfaction; with some resorting to appealing to the royal institutions for help.[33] The evolution in the COVID-19 communication strategy and changes in spokesmen seems to have been an attempt to overcome this distrust.

POLITICAL SPILLOVER ON COVID-19 MANAGEMENT

The issue of distrust affecting COVID-19 communication not only stemmed from deemed incompetency in the political leadership but was also the result of an abundance of fake news that competed with health advisories and updates. KKM tried to dispel this misinformation from the very beginning of the pandemic by posting images of WhatsApp or Facebook messages on their website and social media pages with large *Palsu* (Fake) stamps on them.[34] Tackling and clarifying fake news head on is highly recommended in uncertain times, but the onslaught of misinformation is unrelenting. KKM continues to have to do this until today with all manner of content: miracle cures, relaxations of SOPs, cluster information, etc., as shown in Figure 5.

Distrust in the leadership also occurs because of inconsistencies in officially released information. This also leads to assumptions that official statistics and situation updates are manipulated to enable swift

---

[33] S. Rahman, "Malaysia's King's Role Comes into Sharper Focus as Country Sails Through Bleakest COVID-19 Days Yet", *Channel NewsAsia*, 20 July 2021, https://www.channelnewsasia.com/commentary/malaysia-king-role-sultans-agong-covid-19-parliament-rulers-2046151

[34] https://www.facebook.com/kementeriankesihatanmalaysia/photos/a.10151657414821237/10156689167381237

Figure 5: Images from Kementerian Kesihatan Public Facebook Page Debunking False News

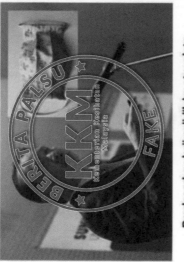

Siasatan dedahkan, pelitup muka fabrik punca kes meningkat

Berdasarkan kaji selidik ke atas data bagaimana pesakit-pesakit ini melaksanakan langkah-langkah perlindungan diri, lebih 75% daripada mereka memaklumkan mereka menggunakan pelitup muka jenis fabrik (washable).

KEMENTERIAN KOMUNIKASI DAN MULTIMEDIA MALAYSIA

PEMAKLUMAN BERITA PALSU

Berikut merupakan **PENAFIAN** tentang berita yang tular di media sosial:

KKM NAFI KES COVID-19 VARIAN OMICRON DI PERAK

Kementerian Kesihatan Malaysia (KKM) **menafikan** kesahihan mesej tular yang mendakwa bahawa varian Omicron yang merupakan varian baharu COVID-19 dengan 32 mutasi 'spike' protein iaitu dua kali ganda lebih banyak daripada varian Delta dikesan di negeri Perak.

KKM **menjelaskan** bahawa setakat ini tiada kes COVID-19 varian Omicron dikesan di Malaysia.

Orang ramai **disaran** agar menghentikan penyebaran maklumat daripada sumber yang tidak sahih yang boleh menimbulkan kebimbangan dan keresahan dalam kalangan masyarakat **sebaliknya** merujuk media sosial rasmi KKM untuk mendapatkan maklumat yang sahih.

Pasukan Respons Pantas
KKMM
30 November 2021 | 10.30 Pagi

Header translations: "Investigation reveals that fabric face masks are the cause of rising infection numbers" (left) and "KKM denies [the existence of] COVID-19 variant Omicron in Perak" (right).

Source: Kementerian Kesihatan Malaysia public Facebook page (18 January 2021 (left) and 30 November 2021 (right)) https://www.facebook.com/37356057236/photos/a.39087994236236/10157650415866237/ (left) and https://www.facebook.com/photo/?fbid=264852739010070&set=a.22189093972917 (right)

economic recovery or further personal goals. On several occasions, there seemed to be conflicting messages from the Prime Minister's Office and DG Noor Hisham.

In July 2021 the Prime Minister announced that more states could transition to Phase 2,[35] and that the National Recovery Plan was on the right track because of increases in daily vaccinations.[36] Positive noises were also made by other ministers on approaching relaxations of MCO restrictions. In contrast, the health ministry was quoted to have warned the government to not be too hasty in relaxing restrictions.[37] DG Noor Hisham again took to his Facebook page to warn about the impending collapse of the healthcare system as a result of the rising numbers of patients needing care in the Intensive Care Unit (ICU).[38]

Photos of doctors treating patients on corridor floors and carparks in several Kuala Lumpur hospitals surfaced on frontliners' personal Facebook pages and myriad news media.[39] DG Noor Hisham was also quoted in mainstream media on the dire situation that hospitals faced.[40]

---

[35] T. Tan, "More States Showing Improvement, May Transition to Phase 2 Soon, Tweets PM from Hospital", *Star Online*, 5 July 2021, https://www.thestar.com.my/news/nation/2021/07/05/more-states-showing-improvement-may-transition-to-phase-2-soon-tweets-pm-from-hospital

[36] M. Nik Anis, "PM: With Daily Vaccinations Crossing 300,000 Doses, National Recovery Plan on the Right Track", *Star Online*, 6 July 2021, https://www.thestar.com.my/news/nation/2021/07/06/pm-with-daily-vaccinations-crossing-300000-doses-national-recovery-plan-on-the-right-track

[37] E. Ng, "Malaysia's Health Ministry Advises Against Easing Curbs Amidst Record-High COVID-19 Cases", *Straits Times*, 6 August 2021, https://www.straitstimes.com/asia/se-asia/malaysias-health-ministry-advised-against-relaxing-restrictions-amid-record-covid-19

[38] Refer to DG Noor Hisham's Facebook post, https://www.facebook.com/DGHisham/photos/pcb.4621735911183594/4621735794516939/

[39] A. Zainudin, "Klang Valley Hospitals on Brink of Collapse", *Code Blue*, 7 July 2021, https://codeblue.galencentre.org/2021/07/07/klang-valley-hospitals-on-the-brink-of-collapse/

[40] *Free Malaysia Today*, "Health Systems on the Brink of Collapse, Says DG", 7 July 2021, https://www.freemalaysiatoday.com/category/nation/2021/07/07/health-systems-on-the-brink-of-collapse-says-dg/

However, Muhyiddin Yassin made a public visit to one of the hospitals in question and media photos showed that the earlier viral images were no longer valid. While accusations arose of the hospital clearing out its Emergency and Trauma ward to move patients to a Trainee Doctors' Dormitory in time for the visit,[41] the claim was debunked by the hospital. Instead, they clarified that they had simply put into place pre-approved plans to expand their treatment wards given the influx of COVID-19 patients.

The viral threads suggesting an alternative truth with regards to the actual pandemic situation indicate the level of distrust that exists in political COVID-19 communication and publicity.

Countless U-turns have also confused and confounded citizens. In May 2021, under the PN government, all sporting activities were banned during MCO 3.0, including outdoor individual sports. This was despite global healthcare recommendations for people to exercise for better mental and physical health in stressful times. The Deputy Minister of Youth and Sport at the time defended the ban as necessary to prevent COVID-19 spread, but later that same day, the minister of the same ministry said that non-contact outdoor recreational sport would be allowed, with SOPs.[42]

Reversals of myriad restrictions throughout the many different stages of MCO have left people bewildered, especially now that there are different recovery phases for different states. This has resulted in citizens either purposely flouting restrictions (many were seen cycling in large groups even though there was still a ban on it) or claiming to have misunderstood the differences in restrictions between states.

While the consequences of breaching outdoor exercise restrictions might be minimal, this example is but the tip of the iceberg in the number

---

[41] *Sun Daily*, "HTAR Denies Claims Emergency and Trauma Dept Vacated Due to PM's Visit", 14 July 2021, https://www.thesundaily.my/home/htar-denies-claims-emergency-and-trauma-dept-vacated-due-to-pm-s-visit-BF8061276

[42] *Malaysiakini* "U-turn: Some Outdoor Sports Allowed in MCO Areas Tomorrow", 7 May 2021, https://www.malaysiakini.com/news/573830

of inconsistencies and U-turns issued by the government throughout the pandemic. Such inconsistencies result in poor control of citizen behaviour and non-compliance with more vital restrictions, which then affects national pandemic recovery.

Another key problem in ensuring compliance with COVID-19 SOPs is fairness disparity. This occurs when political personalities or the wealthy are seen to be able to flout SOPs with little consequences other than "an investigation into reports of non-compliance", but ordinary people are slapped with hefty fines with no questions asked.[43] On the ground, regular people then refuse to abide by SOPs in simple retaliation to the deemed injustices, regardless of the possible effects that it might have on their personal health and safety.

Infighting between or within political parties also hampers pandemic recovery action as politicians resist taking the harsh steps required to stamp out the virus. Given Prime Minister Muhyiddin's questionable takeover of government and precarious position, he needed to pander to his benefactors, the electorate and other ministers to shore up support. A government in need of financial and political endorsement will opt for expedient options, such as acceding to demands by influential business entities (or financial backers) to keep economic sectors open, capitulating to other politicians' requests in return for their backing, or to reduce restrictions to appease a population tired of being kept at home.[44]

As the Coronavirus pandemic is an unprecedented calamity, the government often seemed like it really had no clue what to do. To an extent, this is not unexpected given the Catch-22 situation. Opening up the economy and easing restrictions help with citizens' financial and mental health, but can be disastrous for physical health. As has been seen

---

[43] S. Rahman, "COVID-19 Measures in Malaysia: Resentment and Rancour Brewing on the Ground", *Fulcrum.sg*, 27 May 2021, https://fulcrum.sg/covid-19-measures-in-malaysia-resentment-and-rancour-brewing-on-the-ground/

[44] A. Tayeb, "Political Infighting Hampers Malaysia's Fight against COVID-19", *East Asia Forum*, 24 June 2021, https://www.eastasiaforum.org/2021/06/24/political-infighting-hampers-malaysias-fight-against-covid-19/

since, even vaccinations are not a guarantee of COVID-19 immunity. The less experienced politicians at the helm did not seem to have the necessary capabilities to manage the situation and offered inconsistent messages depending on their ministry or personal interests.

A lack of unity across political divides and between factions within the same party can also hamper cohesive action for pandemic spread. As opposition politicians disagreed with every step taken by the existing regime, party members might also revolt against restrictions.[45] For example, in July 2021 Pakatan Harapan called for Muhyiddin Yassin to step down on account of his failure to control the pandemic and confusing SOPs.[46] UMNO, which is part of Muhyiddin's Perikatan Nasional (PN) coalition also withdrew their support for him at about the same time, also citing his mismanagement of COVID-19.[47] Citizens' desperation and the general view that politicians are not genuinely concerned about the needs of the people result in even weaker government control of the crisis narrative and SOP compliance.

The extent of inclusivity that exists in a country is also a factor that affects successful pandemic communication and response.[48] Malaysia is a country of hundreds of ethnicities and languages, but COVID-19 communication was largely in English and Malay. This excluded minority communities such as those who speak Tamil, Mandarin or other Chinese dialects. The indigenous people were also affected by this lack of consideration; activists and researchers rushed to translate COVID-19 information into indigenous languages to be disseminated through more accessible communication media such as WhatsApp and TikTok. In

---

[45] Lilleker et al. eds., *Political Communication and COVID-19*, p. 7.

[46] T.A. Yusof, "PH Presidential Council Again Calls for PM to Step Down", *New Straits Times*, 10 July 2021, https://www.nst.com.my/news/politics/2021/07/706871/ph-presidential-council-again-calls-pm-step-down

[47] *Al Jazeera*, "Malaysia Party Withdraws Support for Muhyiddin, Citing COVID-19", 8 July 2021, https://www.aljazeera.com/news/2021/7/8/malaysia-party-withdraws-support-for-muhyiddin-amid-covid-surge

[48] Lilleker et al. eds., *Political Communication and COVID-19*, p. 7.

contrast, Singapore's Ministry of Health provided pandemic resources in the four official languages of English, Mandarin, Malay and Tamil.[49]

Beyond social fissures along class, connections, and wealth is the issue of whether all residents are seen as equally eligible for vaccinations. The announcement by the Ministry of Trade and Industry (MITI) that factories must foot the bill for additional costs incurred in vaccinating their workers (even though vaccines are free)[50] indicated that migrant workers were not provided entirely equitable access to vaccines. Instead, their health and safety were in the hands of their employers. That many were unable to get vaccinated became evident in the long desperate queues that emerged when walk-in vaccination centres opened for non-citizens in the Klang Valley.[51]

Given migrant workers' working and living conditions, they are a prime festering ground for the COVID-19 virus. Their exclusion from the national vaccination programme reduces the effectiveness of pandemic recovery efforts.[52] This was made worse by the immigration department's raids on overstayers, irregular migrants and the stateless as they tried to get vaccinated.[53]

---

[49] Ministry of Health Singapore website, "Content You Can Use", https://www.moh.gov.sg/covid-19/general/resources (accessed 30 November 2021).

[50] C. Lee, "Malaysian Companies Must Shoulder Additional Costs for Vaccination", HRMasia website, 15 June 2021, https://hrmasia.com/companies-must-shoulder-additional-costs-for-workers-vaccination-says-malaysian-government/

[51] *Straits Times*, "Viral Video of 'Hugging Queues' for COVID-19 Vaccine in Malaysia Sparks Outcry", 12 August 2021, https://www.straitstimes.com/asia/se-asia/viral-video-of-hugging-queue-in-malaysia-for-covid-19-vaccine-sparks-outcry

[52] N. Muhamad Noor, and Y.S. Loong, "COVID-19: The Case for Vaccinating Migrants, too", Khazanah Research Institute, 25 January 2021, http://www.krinstitute.org/Views-@-Covid-19-;_The_Case_for_Vaccinating_Migrants,_Too.aspx

[53] Human Rights Watch, "Malaysia: Raids on Migrants Hinder Vaccine Access", 30 June 2021, https://www.hrw.org/news/2021/06/30/malaysia-raids-migrants-hinder-vaccine-access

ANALYSING MALAYSIA'S PANDEMIC COMMUNICATION CONTENT

The following section will take a closer look at the content disseminated by the Ministry of Health throughout the pandemic and assess how effective it has been based on the framework provided earlier.

Clarity, Simplicity and Accessibility

From the outset, KKM provided its audiences with clear, simple, and accessible infographics with advice on what to do to prevent infection. In the early days, focus seemed to be on showing how many COVID-19 cases there were worldwide, and in comparison, how few there were in Malaysia.[54] Most infographics then had specific advice on what to do. However, as information on the virus was sparse, this focused on not touching wild animals or eating raw meat. Frequent hand washing was recommended but masks were not yet deemed vital or mandatory. While these infographics were available, most of the posts on KKM's Facebook page were word- and statistics-heavy press releases from relevant government ministries.[55]

With the first cases of COVID-19 arriving in Malaysia through tourists from China, the emphasis at the time was focused on stressing that the "Wuhan Coronavirus" needed to be (and could be) stopped at international entry points. The first few photos that did not feature leaders on publicity rounds showed HAZMAT (hazardous materials) teams greeting tourists from China on the airport tarmac, fully decked out in protective gear and redirecting them to testing and isolation facilities.[56]

---

[54] https://www.facebook.com/kementeriankesihatanmalaysia/photos/a.10151657414821237/10156683783991237

[55] https://www.facebook.com/kementeriankesihatanmalaysia/photos/a.10151657414821237/10156686877376237

[56] https://www.facebook.com/kementeriankesihatanmalaysia/photos/a.10151657414821237/10156712944006237

This imagery was one of chemical warfare and defence, and included photos of medical and HAZMAT response teams gearing up and saying prayers[57] before shepherding disembarking tourists, including women and young children, into the airport building.[58] These seemed to show that the government had everything under control, and extreme precautions were being taken to keep the country safe from an external threat.

Using Narrative Persuasion for Behavioural Change

Narrative persuasion is highly recommended in communicating crises, as people are more likely to amend their behaviour out of concern for the welfare of others instead of through the negative instigation of fear.[59] Fear of infection, however, leads people to look for more information. In the early days of the pandemic, a lack of reliable information led to increased sensitivity to widely abundant misinformation and conspiracy theories (especially given the early lack of proven facts on COVID-19), and subsequently the swift spread of fake news.[60]

The KKM Facebook page first applied the narrative persuasion approach after the first COVID-19 deaths occurred in March 2020. This also coincided with MCO 1.0 and the closing of national borders. Frontliners (including pregnant nurses and doctors) were featured holding signs appealing to people to stay home while they stayed at work to deal

---

[57] https://www.facebook.com/kementeriankesihatanmalaysia/photos/a.10151657414821237/10156712944511237

[58] https://www.facebook.com/kementeriankesihatanmalaysia/photos/a.10151657414821237/10156774236461237

[59] E.B. Hester, B. Ivanov, and K.A. Parker, "Overcoming Obstacles to Collective Action by Communicating Compassion in Science", in *Communicating Science in Times of Crisis*, edited by O'Hair and O'Hair, p. 155.

[60] C. Salvi, P. Iannello, A. Cancer, M. McClay, S. Rago, J.E. Dunsmoor, and A. Antonietti, "Going Viral: How Fear, Socio-Cognitive Polarization and Problem-Solving Influence Fake News Detection and Proliferation During Covid-19 Pandemic", *Frontiers in Communication*, 12 January 2021, https://doi.org/10.3389/fcomm.2020.562588

with the virus.[61] This approach highlighted the sacrifices that frontliners were making, while pleading for others to do their part (by staying home) to fight the pandemic.

At the end of March 2020, as deaths continued to rise, this compassionate appeal was used again in a post featuring frontliners clad in protective personal equipment (PPE) hugging each other in sorrow as KKM announced yet another death (the fifteenth in all cumulative deaths at the time) related to the Sri Petaling religious cluster.[62]

A photo displaying the suffering of frontliners[63] or pointed photos of ICU conditions, death, and burial,[64] might elicit compassion and a sense of having to do something to help the plight of both medical staff and patients. While DG Noor Hisham first posted images of COVID-19 deaths in January 2021,[65] these were reposted from international images and hence may not have been as effective in instigating local action or behavioural change. Viewers often struggle to make the connection when the images or footage used is not personalized or "close to home".

He also shared images from the Johor Department of Health depicting PPE-clad undertakers preparing coffins for COVID-19 burials.[66] While

[61] https://www.facebook.com/kementeriankesihatanmalaysia/photos/a.10151657414821237/10156834812126237

[62] https://www.facebook.com/kementeriankesihatanmalaysia/photos/a.10151657414821237/10156845896151237

[63] As posted by DG Noor Hisham on his Facebook page, https://www.facebook.com/DGHisham/posts/4410998348924019

[64] An example of what may have been a more convincing post is shown in H. Hazlin, "'Photos of Bodies Stacked at Hospital Are Real': Malaysia's Undertakers Struggle as COVID-19 Deaths Soar", *Straits Times*, 30 July 2021, https://www.straitstimes.com/asia/se-asia/undertakers-work-round-the-clock-in-malaysia-as-covid-19-deaths-soar

[65] Refer to DG Noor Hisham's Facebook page, https://www.facebook.com/DGHisham/photos/pcb.3990363417654183/3990363254320866/

[66] Refer to DG Noor Hisham's Facebook page, https://www.facebook.com/jabatankesihatannegerijohor/photos/pcb.3665788090135113/36657721868 03370

this elicited more worried responses, it still does not have as much impact as watching PPE-clad undertakers burying or cremating the dead,[67] or footage of a hearse driving slowly past a house for the family to wave farewell for the last time.[68]

The KKM Facebook page was also slow to post images of local death and burial, but a more effective approach would have been the dissemination of short videos of burials or frontliners' preparations for burial via WhatsApp or TikTok. While this returns to negative persuasion methods, the dire situation and the advent of more accurate information (compared to the early days of the pandemic) may have driven home the need for more precautions given the severity of the situation, especially when dispersed by more widely used media. While there may be privacy issues related to this, there are myriad ways to mask identity, and such public service announcements (PSAs) might have been more effective in convincing rural communities of the immediate dangers of COVID-19.

Private individuals and organizations have on many occasions created and disseminated images and videos discouraging people to return to their rural villages for festive seasons to prevent the spread of COVID-19.[69] Given the exponential rise in cases in the first half of 2021, local media began to take the first step to show photos of COVID-19-burials, regardless of cultural taboos or sensitivities.[70]

[67] Kinilens, "Of COVID-19 and Cremation of the Dead", *Malaysiakini*, 2021, https://www.malaysiakini.com/photos/578992

[68] T.N. Alagesh, "Heartbreak, as Slow-Moving Hearse Allows Family to Bid Final Adieu to Late Mother", *New Straits Times*, 5 July 2021, https://www.nst.com.my/news/nation/2021/07/705357/heartbreak-slow-moving-hearse-allows-family-bid-final-adieu-late-mother

[69] FINAS, "FINAS Raya 2020: Jangan Balik Kampung!", 21 May 2020, https://www.youtube.com/watch?v=dqJS-2SUgxQ

[70] R. Maelzer, "Coronavirus Pandemic: Malaysia Sees Record COVID-19 Cases, Deaths", CGTN, 21 May 2021, https://news.cgtn.com/news/2021-05-21/VHJhbnNjcmlwdDU0OTATAx/index.html

Segmenting Audiences for Effective Messaging

As the situation worsened, KKM's posts included colourful maps that effectively illustrated infection locations and numbers.[71] These early maps also had specific instructions on how to keep the virus out of neighbourhoods and communities. This however seemed to reinforce the initial perception that COVID-19 was an urban problem, and that rural communities were safe from its threat.

The Risk Perception Attitude Framework[72] recommends segmenting audiences based on their risk bias. Rural communities which struggle to grasp the severity of the pandemic, either because it is seen as a distant intangible threat or because they feel physically isolated from the risks[73] need specially targeted messages to ensure that they understand the dangers.

The language used needs to be accessible in terms of simplicity and inclusive so as to reach all ethnicities. As prescribed in terror management theory, worst-case scenarios need to be clearly depicted for a disbelieving audience. Risk communication strategies[74] also recommend highlighting potential yet unseen negative consequences for areas that have not yet been affected by the virus—before it reaches their communities.

Much of the information on the KKM Facebook page and website are quite technical. There is a lot of information on the virus, as well

---

[71] https://www.facebook.com/kementeriankesihatanmalaysia/photos/a.10151657414821237/10156877334261237 and https://www.facebook.com/kementeriankesihatanmalaysia/photos/a.10151657414821237/10156877334276237

[72] Real et al., "Communication and COVID-19: Challenges in Evidence-Based Healthcare Design", in *Communicating Science in Times of Crisis*, edited by O'Hair and O'Hair, p. 85.

[73] K.B. Wright, "Social Media, Risk Perceptions Related to COVID-19, and Health Outcomes", in *Communicating Science in Times of Crisis*, edited by O'Hair and O'Hair, p. 130.

[74] Real et al., "Communication and COVID-19: Challenges in Evidence-Based Healthcare Design", in *Communicating Science in Times of Crisis*, edited by O'Hair and O'Hair, p. 88.

as statistics, graphs and numbers. In the early stages of a new crisis like Coronavirus, more information may be welcome as people seek answers to an unprecedented situation. However, as time passes and the crisis deepens over a longer period, readers and viewers become numb to the figures and it all becomes information overload as the statistics overwhelm processing capacities. This is especially evident when pandemic fatigue sets in.[75]

Communication strategies must then switch to appeal on a more emotional level at this stage, as well as more easily digestible bytes of information and infographics that everyone can comprehend regardless of language or education level. In mid-2021, KKM began to introduce more useful information that conveyed the percentage of new infections in the more dangerous categories of infection, as well as percentages in ICU as shown in Figure 6. This provides a clearer understanding of the severity of the situation than merely high numbers of infection, which may include milder, less dangerous infections.

However, for rural, indigenous, or less educated populations that may not be able to process too much text, numbers or statistics, much of the information dissemination held no meaning from the beginning. While infographics were colourful, with some in Malay and simple words, they were not effective in conveying the severity of the threat they faced. Also given the tendency for rural communities to depend on WhatsApp, Telegram or TikTok as a means of communication, the message medium is also important. This underlines why segmenting messages to cater to different recipient groups, and using channels that appeal to the various segments, may have been a more effective strategy.

Similar ineffectiveness occurred in the communication of the need for vaccines. While there was also the additional factor of fake news that debunked the safety and efficacy of vaccines, there also seemed to be a lack of understanding of how to convey the need for vaccines to (especially)

---

[75] J.W. Muhamad, and P. Merle, "Identity and Information Overload: Examining the Impact of Health Messaging in Times of Crisis", in *Communicating Science in Times of Crisis*, edited by O'Hair and O'Hair, p. 113.

***Figure 6: Example of the Ministry of Health Malaysia's
COVID-19 Communication Infographic: Infections by
Category***

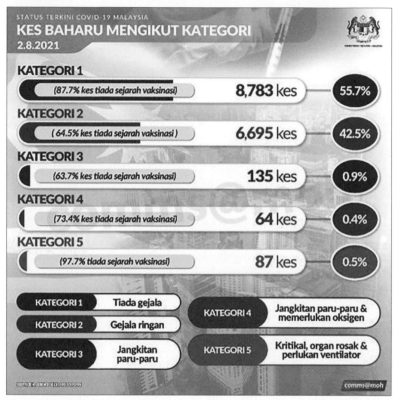

Note: This type of infographic was also posted daily on the main KKM Facebook
page until the regime change and the installation of Khairy Jamaluddin as
Minister of Health.
Source: Ministry of Health Malaysia website, 2 August 2021, https://covid-19.
moh.gov.my/terkini/2021/08/situasi-terkini-covid-19-di-malaysia-02082021

rural, indigenous, and other B40 (bottom 40 per cent) communities. Evidence of this ranged from political parties putting up banners that did not consider local sensitivities and biases, to some religious leaders injecting doubt over the severity of the virus by championing the belief that fear of God is more important than fear of a virus.[76]

As the pandemic situation got worse and the epicentre of the infection spread beyond the Klang Valley to other more rural states, infection, illness, and deaths became the daily reality for many communities. Witnessing the severity of the virus first-hand has since encouraged more rural, indigenous and B40 communities to overcome vaccine hesitancy. This was coupled with more efforts by KKM to mobilize volunteers and healthcare workers into communities to engage with the doubtful, and bring vaccines to rural areas in mobile vaccination vehicles. With an increase of vaccine availability for states beyond the Klang Valley, several walk-in vaccination centres opened in suburban townships, and this too helped to boost vaccination numbers.

Indigenous activists, civil society organizations and personnel from the Indigenous Peoples' Hospital, Gombak (Hospital Orang Asli Gombak, or HOAG) were also on the ground to convince indigenous communities about the severity of COVID-19, its reach, and the need for vaccination. Commands by the royal houses to get vaccinated (or possibly lose jobs) also played a role in encouraging people to overcome vaccine-hesitancy. Announced easing of restrictions for the vaccinated were also crucial in forcing the unwilling to get vaccinated as many were eager to be released from extended COVID-induced confinement.

Perhaps if more of these efforts had been applied from the very beginning of the pandemic, there may have been less infection and spread to rural areas at the end of 2020. Table 4 summarizes the analysis of KKM's communication strategy and provides suggestions for improvements in relation to the ideal communication aspects highlighted in the earlier sections.

---

[76] H. Beech, "'None of Us Have a Fear of Corona': The Faithful at an Outbreak's Centre", *New York Times*, 20 March 2020, https://www.nytimes.com/2020/03/20/world/asia/coronavirus-malaysia-muslims-outbreak.html

Table 4: Summary Analysis of Malaysia's Official COVID-19 Communication Strategy

	Ideal Communication Features	Evaluation	Suggestions
1	Clear, simple and accessible	☑ infographics and maps ⊗ some graphs and figures are difficult for the layman to decipher ⊗ after a while there is statistical overload ✪ *with the latest regime change:* some of the previous information is no longer available; statistics are not updated as often; information is less appealing and inaccessible	◉ use more emotive photographs and short video clips ◉ use more of the local languages (Malay, Tamil, Mandarin or dialects) ◉ retain maps, cluster information and colour in infographics ◉ add accessible explanations to complicated graphics and statistics ◉ return to past approach to sharing, updating, and collecting data
2	Flexible strategy to meet evolving situation	☑ politician or expert-prominence models of communication evolved based on existing political situation and public responses ⊗ communication content did not evolve to meet the needs of the day (e.g., to overcome information overload)	◉ return to original purpose of disseminating important health information ◉ balance statistical information with appealing infographics/photos/videos that provide useful advice as the COVID-19 situation changes

continued on next page

#			
	✪ *with the latest regime change: focus seems to be more on political popularity than disseminating necessary information*		◉ as the situation worsens, use strong imagery and footage of ICU wards, masked patients (to avoid identification) suffering or offering testimonials and their negative experiences, and isolated COVID-19 burials where the family is unable to be present during the patient's last moments
3	Tackles and clarifies misinformation	☑ KKM has been consistently doing this on its Facebook and website since Day 1 ⊗ There continues to be strong anti-vax and pro-Ivermectin groups who consistently produce a counter-narrative to KKM's information	◉ Fake news clarifications also need to be disseminated by WhatsApp and TikTok to reach rural communities ◉ Provide some alternative information that counters folk cures or provides positive traditional remedies to reduce COVID-19 symptoms and discomfort or increase resilience (e.g., increase Vitamin C intake, drink coconut water, etc.)
4	Suggest action for behavioural change with benefits to self	☑ infographics have clear instructions on what to do ⊗ infographics do not always provide the *why* (this can sometimes counter fake news claims)	◉ use emotional and compassionate appeals to ensure useful action and behavioural change

Table 4 — cont'd

	Ideal Communication Features	Evaluation	Suggestions
5	Suit message to segmented audience	☑ abundant information for those who needed facts, statistics and figures ☑ posts and messages are in English and Bahasa Malaysia ☑ KKM offers myriad talks by doctors to explain COVID-19 and its related issues ☑ KKM has gone to the ground to engage with vaccine-hesitant communities and launched mobile vaccination centres to reach rural communities ⊗ posts do not appeal to rural, less educated or indigenous communities ⊗ minority languages were excluded in official messaging ⊗ not everyone has access to Zoom or GoogleMeet to listen to webinars	◉ add posts in other local languages or dialects, including indigenous languages ◉ use other media channels with simpler, more direct content that reaches rural and indigenous communities (radio, WhatsApp, TikTok) ◉ work closely with Jabatan Kemajuan Orang Asli (JAKOA), civil society organizations and religious authorities with existing networks on the ground to disseminate accurate information, encourage vaccination and debunk fake news ◉ acknowledge limitations among the B40 community with regards to being able to rest for an extended period post-vaccination; to work from home and offer alternative solutions
6	Consistent, credible and reliable	⊗ has not been successful because of political machinations and unstable government	◉ provide one point of reliable, credible source of information (such as DG Noor Hisham)

GRASSROOTS COVID-19 COMMUNICATION

Throughout the pandemic, numerous individuals and groups have taken it upon themselves to disseminate COVID-19-related information to their networks. While some of these pages and groups on Facebook were created specifically for the pandemic period, others are just sharing information that they deemed useful to their audiences.[77] Two examples worth highlighting as increasingly popular sources of information are the Gerai OA and OA Lindungi Komuniti Facebook pages.[78]

Gerai OA is a Facebook page run by indigenous craft expert Reita Rahim. It has been in existence for more than a decade and was originally created to promote and sell indigenous products, but eventually evolved to also raise funds and support for indigenous needs and other issues. Due to a number of national disasters, however, the page has taken to providing its audience with pertinent information and updates that may not be easily available from other sources. Some of these earlier incidents included the Mount Kinabalu earthquake and severe flooding events, especially when they affected indigenous communities.

During COVID-19, Gerai OA updated its largely English-reading audiences with explanations of the latest pandemic news; it also highlighted statistics that mattered the most, and COVID-19 impacts on indigenous communities. The Facebook page also untangled contrary announcements from myriad political personalities and clarified confusing SOPs. While some posts are lengthy clarifications, statistical explanations and political discussions, others are short and impactful such as shown in Figure 7.

---

[77] The following pages are examples of those focused mainly on Johor audiences (many of whom were directly affected by the COVID-19-induced Singapore-Johor border closure), who adapted their content to include COVID-19 information: Makmur Johor, JB Tracer and Southern Vengers.

[78] OA is an abbreviation for Orang Asli (referring to the indigenous people of Peninsular Malaysia) or Orang Asal (indigenous people of both East and West Malaysia). Orang Asli thus fall under Orang Asal, but in these abbreviated forms, OA can refer to either, or both.

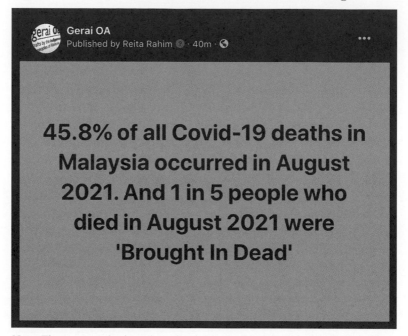

Note: The post emphasizes the spike in deaths in Malaysia, information that is not easily found or written as pointedly on the Ministry of Health's website or Facebook pages.

Source: Reproduced with permission from Gerai OA.

Figure 7 was posted at a time when COVID-related death information was only referred to indirectly, hidden by statistics and numbers that are often beyond the general processing ability of the average layman audience. The post is just one example of how Gerai OA provided succinct and reliable (meticulously fact-checked) information to encourage people to take action to reduce the spread of COVID-19. Many of the page's followers have applauded Gerai OA volunteers for their ability to simplify highly complicated political machinations, digest and summarize politicians' pandemic speeches, as well as make sense of often overlapping and arbitrary restrictions. This Facebook page has become the go-to site for those trying to understand current pandemic conditions beyond the propaganda and hubris of government pages.

OA Lindungi Komuniti is a Facebook page that was created during the pandemic to specifically provide COVID-19-related information to the indigenous community. Created by an academic-cum-indigenous activist, Dr Rusaslina Idrus, the page has been extremely active in posting accessible, engaging and shareable posters on COVID-19 in myriad indigenous languages. Most recently, it held a short video competition to encourage the creation of content that can be easily shared by indigenous communities on WhatsApp and TikTok to debunk fake news and spread accurate virus information.[79]

This effort is especially effective because the videos are made by indigenous people for other indigenous people. They are then able to combat the fake news of the moment and address the fears and uncertainties faced by their communities. Having an indigenous person as the narrator and speaking in a familiar language, makes the content more accessible, trustworthy and convincing, especially when there is a history of distrust of government medical authorities.

The difference between both these pages and official government pages (especially KKM) is the former's ability to assess, understand and meet the information needs of their followers. They fill a gap left empty by the authorities and play a huge role in ensuring that vital COVID-19 information reaches their audiences. This is key to ensuring public compliance with COVID-19 restrictions and instigating behavioural change to reduce infections.

THE FUTURE OF COVID-19 COMMUNICATION

With the appointment of Khairy Jamaluddin as Minister of Health, a new KKM website promising more accessible and easy-to-understand

---

[79] I. Lim, "Malaysia's Orang Asli Get Creative with TikTok, Posters, WhatsApp Audio to Promote COVID-19 SOPs, Vaccination", *Malay Mail*, 4 September 2021, https://www.malaymail.com/amp/news/malaysia/2021/09/04/malaysias-orang-asli-get-creative-with-tiktok-posters-whatsapp-audio-to-pro/2002852

COVID-19 data was launched.[80] A GitHub site (https://github.com/MoH-Malaysia) that provides raw COVID-19-related data that was launched under the previous regime continues to exist as a publicly accessible source.

However, since the launch of the CovidNOW website, some of the older infographics that many had grown reliant on, such as cluster information and maps, as well as death rate and infection percentages are no longer posted on the KKM Facebook page. Instead, this information has to be dug up from the CovidNOW and GitHub sites. Unfortunately, the infographics have now lost their visual appeal, using less colour and smaller font. The GitHub site is not updated daily as it was under the previous regime, meaning that data is dated, and even harder to find. Numerous complaints about the changes have been posted in KKM Facebook page comments, to the point where the commenting option was turned off for some posts.

While this evolution might be the inadvertent result of Khairy Jamaluddin's assumed popularity, it has made the sourcing of information more difficult. Questions have arisen over whether the lag in updating data and missing information is an intentional step to conceal the actual state of the pandemic in order to endorse the loosening of restrictions and reopening of the economy, or if it is just oversight and a complete misunderstanding of the public's information needs.

The KKM Facebook page now seems to be posting more photographs of the new Minister of Health on his publicity rounds, and his public announcements. DG Noor Hisham seems to be less visible, except when he is quoted in the media with a warning on rising infectivity rates or other bad news.[81]

---

[80] Astro Awani,"MOH Launches New COVID-19 Data Website", 9 September 2021, https://www.astroawani.com/berita-malaysia/moh-launches-new-covid19-data-website-318896

[81] Refer to S.J. Zahiid, "Health DG Warns of Rising COVID-19 Infectivity Even as More Malaysians Are Vaccinated", *Yahoo News*, 17 November 2021, https://malaysia.news.yahoo.com/health-dg-warns-rising-covid-014936375.html and *Malay Mail*, "COVID-19: 84 Cases Detected During Current Parliament Sitting, Says Dr Noor Hisham", 30 November 2021, https://www.malaymail.com/news/malaysia/2021/11/30/covid-19-84-cases-detected-during-current-parliament-sitting-says-dr-noor-h/2024959

As the pandemic continues, a balance needs to be found between providing accurate data that assuages public concerns and answers questions, and also employs a compelling narrative to ensure that the public adopts proper precautions to prevent COVID-19 spread. There is still so much uncertainty about the pandemic, its vaccines, and any possible cure, as well as the probability that new variants such as Omicron could wreak worse damage on the population, especially with both the economy and borders gradually reopening. It is thus vital that the government employs a holistic communication approach as described above.

The only way that Malaysia can overcome this health crisis is for its politicians and people to come together to do what is necessary—and this can only be done with sufficient, accurate, transparent, and reliable information.